Four Quadrant Easy Diet Plan

Robert Stetson

Four Quadrant Easy Diet Plan
Copyright 2016 By Robert Stetson
ALL RIGHTS RESERVED

INTRODUCTION

Since I am neither a Physician, nor a nutritionist, legal prudence suggests that none of the advice in this book is intended as medical advice.

It is imperative that you seek the advice of your healthcare professional regarding any of the suggestions given here.

This dietary practice has worked for me, but may not be right for everyone.

This weight control process is the product of a frustrated diabetic who found success in a pain free weight control method.

Try as you might, dieting is one of the most difficult tasks to complete. Stop dieting and eliminate the phycology of breakfast, lunch and dinner. Meals need not have names.

Maintaining your newly achieved target weight becomes possible without ongoing difficulty.

This is not a diet. It is a weight control process. It successfully addresses the pain of weight loss and maintenance.

Two factors govern your levels of hunger and loss.

1. Carbs and calories vs. Blood sugar levels.
2. The painful hunger curve that tries our souls.

The hunger curve is determined by the time between meals. If you dine at 6 PM and your next meal is at 6 AM, you're going to need a "snack" at midnight. This leads to nibbling on chips and popcorn, etc.

This new approach to weight loss eliminates the "fast" in "breakfast" and allows you the comfort of four meals a day, evenly spaced and satisfying.

Follow this new approach to weight loss and weight management where meals do not have names.

This approach eliminates the evening craving stretch, where snacking does you in.

This approach also eliminates the elusive mystery of how to lose weight and how to keep it off.

TABLE OF CONTENTS

THE QUADRANT METHOD

It is imperative that you seek the advice of your healthcare professional regarding any of the suggestions given here.

This dietary practice has worked for me, but may not be right for everyone.

This weight control process is the product of a frustrated diabetic who found success in a pain free weight control method.

Traditional diet and weight control plans have you eating three meals a day and then fasting from after dinner (the evening meal), to breakfast. This is why the morning meal is called "break-fast".

This book breaks the cycle of mealtime stereotypes and offers a whole new flexibility with regard to what you choose to eat and when.

If you have ever awakened and had a hankering for a good steak, potato and vegetable, you are not alone. The desire for a good steak in the morning was probably the beginning of the steak and eggs idea.

Many times, at 7 PM, I would want a breakfast.

My friends look at me and ask, "Breakfast at this hour?" I do not understand the question. Let's stop naming our meals and get down to making mealtime more enjoyable. To this end,

II have named a chapter in this book, "No More Meal Labels".

Do not fast! Proper weight control does not encourage fasting, as this can lead to improper diet and subsequently, binge eating. You will be far more successful with managing your weight when you are never hungry.

Weight loss is always made easier in the "never hungry" environment.

The quadrant method allows you to go to bed immediately after eating a meal. If you cannot sleep well after eating a meal, you can redistribute the missing calories to other meals. It is your choice.

Your weight changes are going to be amazing at times. Usually in the beginning.

Your weight changes are going to be slow at times. Once your body realizes that it needs to conserve energy.

Your weight changes are going to be plateaued at times. When your body digs in its figurative heels and says, "Enough is enough."

The quadrant method allows you to step back and allow the body to accept your new reduced weight as normal. It is OK to establish a beachhead and set up a new perimeter, in a manner of speaking.

Details on how I took the strain off of my progress and allowed me to restart meaningful weight loss again, starting with a lower "set point" is outlined in the chapter, "Rate Management Mode".

You get hungry, mostly at night, because your body has internalized the habit of fasting from 6 PM to 6 AM. Twelve hours is a long time when you already feel that you haven't had enough to eat. The Quadrant Method fixes that problem.

The appropriate method for determining the number of calories per meal is to take your total daily caloric intake target and divide by 4. In the event that your caloric intake is 1800 calories per day, your daily meals would equal 450. If you were on a 1200 or 1500 calorie weight loss plan, then the meals would equal 300 or 375 respectively.

Cravings and binge eating are less likely, especially if you have an addictive personality.

The quadrant method works even better when you adopt the attitude where meals have no name. Forget about breakfast, lunch, dinner, supper and snacks. A meal is a meal, nothing more, nothing less.

You can glean from this plan description, that snacks are not allowed. The key is a more even caloric distribution.

If you are diabetic, the counting of carbohydrates is extremely important. It allows you to track and otherwise control your blood sugar levels. Carb counting also enables you to regulate your insulin requirements.

LIFESTYLE VS WEIGHT LOSS

The first thing people think of when they think of lifestyle is the level of exercise and other general physical activity. How mobile are you? Do you work out? Many other questions arise.

You can do strenuous exercises that have sweat dripping from your nose every day and wonder why you are not losing weight. Exercise is beneficial, do not get me wrong.

Exercise can establish a more heightened metabolic rate that continues to burn calories even after the exercise stops. Don't count on exercise to make a dramatic difference by itself. You have more success by reducing you caloric intake far more than trying to burn calories off.

If you exercise, good for you. Keep it up. Try not to slump into a sedentary lifestyle. It will hinder your progress and leave you depressed.

There is a lot of information available regarding lifestyle with regard to exercise. The lifestyle of one who is living on a reduced calorie intake is more complicated than that. It encompasses many factors effecting the general mood and effectiveness of the goal to reduce one's body mass.

Nothing quite attacks the spirit more severely than fads. Specialty delivered meal plans and potions that claim to "make the pounds vanish, as if by magic".

If they do not work and most of them do not work, then they rob you of your money and give you false hope.

If they do work, and I have not found any that do, they do nothing to perpetuate their success. After you abandon the fad, as you must, the pounds reappear, as if by magic.

You cannot maintain that level of stress on your system permanently.

You say, "Ah! What about those magic pills? Those keep you from digesting fat. Yes, they work. The fat goes right through you. Can you say, "Anal seepage"? It ruins your clothes by creating oil stains in the seat of your pants and is embarrassing. This happens when you when you eat something fat or oily, that you should not have eaten.

I once had a Doctor say, when they were attempting to prescribe the fat inhibiting pills, "You shouldn't be eating fat anyway."

I had yet another Doctor say, "Without fat in the diet, you run the risk of gallstones."

My opinion is that, fat is a natural part of any diet and should constitute up to 30% of your calories, as I have been told by, yet another Doctor.

On the other hand, If not eating any fat is the key to losing the weight and not the pills themselves, what do I need the pills for?

It seems that the only purpose the pills really serve, is to punish you while ruining your clothing, should you eat anything you should not.

I should not only dispense with the fat, I should also dispense with the pills.

The digestive system needs fat to function, I am told, because the gall bladder can begin to retain the bile when there is no food to process. This can lead to gallstones and surgery.

We are omnivorous creatures by nature and our systems are designed to process fats as a matter of course, even if it is just vegetable fats.

There is no difference between simple weight control and weight loss. Diet does not mean weight loss. It simply means what you eat and when.

If you are overweight, the problem is not that you are overweight. The problem is with your daily diet. Stop trying to fix the symptom and start fixing the cause.

If you were at your ideal weight tomorrow, you would be right back where you are in no time.

I will help you fix the cause of your problem. Your weight will fix itself and remain fixed.

Focus on your eating habits and be patient. This is going to take a while, but it will be a permanent fix.

This is not a diet in the traditional sense, because it merely establishes the caloric requirement and then distributes the number of daily calories over the course of a day.

This is something you should have always done and will be doing for the rest of your life.

It is not what you eat that is killing you. It's how much you eat. It is not even a matter of when you eat, as much as the total number of calories consumed over the course of any and every 24 hour period.

RATE MANAGEMENT MODE

Look at where you are and ask yourself where you want to be a year from now. I used to become tired of hearing about how long it took to become overweight and how it will take as long to lose it. I wanted instant results, but instant results are not lasting results.

If you woke up tomorrow at your ideal weight, you would not have fixed a thing. You need to correct the situation that created the problem.

Avoid the moaners and the groaners. Do not join diet groups that meet regularly and weigh in. Each person stands up and talks about the agony of dieting. They will only depress and discourage you.

They say things like, "I find myself dreaming about food, like sugarplums dancing in my head".

The next person stands and says, "I broke down and ate a whole pie on Friday last week. I gained back five pounds".

How does this help you? When I was a member of a weight loss group, the weekly meetings left me depressed after listening to all of the horror stories. When you're hungry all of the time, you have problems of your own. I stopped going and lost the weight successfully.

Ignore the problem for now and focus on the situation governing what you eat, how often and how much. The weight problem will fix itself. If you do not start losing weight after a few days, then you have not corrected the problem.

After you lose about 10 to 20 pounds, the weight will stop coming off for a while. This is a plateau and is normal.

When I hit my plateau after 6 months and 25 pounds, I was beside myself. Even knowing its completely normal, the rate at which the weight falls away slows and even stops for a while.

The body has defenses against starvation and will slow many of the body's processes to save on energy and resources. Your hair and nails will even slow their growth.

What I did was risky, but it worked. I took on a few more calories for about 2 weeks. The goal was to trick the body into adjusting to the new weight.

Once the body accepted the new weight, I went back on the lower calorie regimen. By "a few more calories", I mean that I went into maintenance mode for the lower weight I had achieved, being very careful to not put any of the original weight back on.

This was a difficult balancing act, because the body had slowed many of the calorie burning activity and the calorie maintenance intake was a bit lower than the previous weight loss intake.

I gained a couple of pounds in spite of (or because of) my careful monitoring and caloric changes.

Then I snapped back into my aggressive calorie reduced weight loss schedule and once again, I enjoyed an initial surge of weight loss. I was back to having the pounds melt away, all the while knowing, "This too shall pass".

NUTRIENT DISTRIBUTION

While you are managing your diet and enjoying the positive changes that are occurring, remember to monitor the daily diet essentials, such as your intake of nutrients, calories, carbohydrates, protein, minerals and vitamins.

Your daily requirements will vary depending on your weight and level of physical activity. In this book, it will always be assumed that your rate of physical activity is minimal, or nonexistent.

The proportional distribution of fat, protein and carbohydrates will remain the same for everyone. Only the volume will differ.

As your weight loss progresses, you will need to recalculate the number of calories and other nutrients, because your body mass is gradually changing.

The average person's requirement:
Calories 2000
Protein 125 grams (500)
Carbohydrates 250 grams (1000)
Fat 56 grams (500)

These metrics can be used as a guide for our example here. Your numbers will vary depending on your height, weight and the number of total calories burned, based on your level of activity.

Distribution:
Fat: 25% of total calories
Protein: 25% of total calories
Carbohydrates: 50% of total calories

Get out a paper and pencil and start writing down some of the favorite food items and their caloric content. If you do not know what the caloric content of a food item is, consult the nutritional information panel on the package, or look it up on the Internet.

By having foods listed on paper, you need only look at the list to plan a meal that conforms to your caloric goals.

For example:

For a caloric allotment of about 400 calories per meal, you can easily get close by simply assembling ingredients to form the meal.

JUST TRACKING CALORIES?:

Scali Bread, 2 slices	100 calories
Chicken, 3 slices	90 calories
Banana, 1 medium	100 calories
Mayonnaise, 1 TBSP.	105 calories

TOTAL: 395

If you want to go beyond the simple calorie counting method and track the absolute values for the ingredients, the numbers are shown here.

FEELING AMBITIOUS?:

Scali Bread, 2 slices	100 calories
Fat:	0 GRAMS
Protein:	4 GRAMS
Carbohydrates:	20 GRAMS

Chicken, 3 slices	90 calories
Fat:	1.5 GRAMS
Protein:	15 GRAMS
Carbohydrates:	6 GRAMS

Banana, 1 medium	100 calories
Fat:	,4 GRAMS
Protein:	1.5 GRAMS
Carbohydrates:	27 GRAMS

Mayonnaise, 1 TBSP.	105 calories
Fat:	10 GRAMS
Protein:	.1 GRAMS
Carbohydrates:	.1 GRAMS

TOTAL FOR THE MEAL:

Fat:	11.9 GRAMS
Protein:	20.6 GRAMS
Carbohydrates:	47.1 GRAMS

You can see the distribution of the ingredients in our meal conforms to the calorie requirements very nicely. When we check the percentage of distribution for fat, protein and carbohydrates, we are way off.

The fat is only 11.9 grams, but should be around 23.5 grams total. That puts the value at around 25% of the 47.1 value.

The protein is 20.6 grams. Only 3.4 grams off from the 24 gram target. but should be around 23.5 grams total. That puts the value at around 43% of the 47.1 value.

Carbohydrates, at 47.1 grams forms the distribution basis for the other values.

Using this guide, you can create an approximate 400 calorie meal as part of a 1,600 calorie plan easily.

When you have to factor in the proper distribution of the elements, the task becomes sufficiently complex to make it impractical.

This guide has enabled you to make a meal of a chicken sandwich with a banana as a healthy desert. If you want coffee or other beverage, you can list the caloric content of your creamer, sweetener other beverage. I usually enjoy a flavorful glass of water with a zero calorie flavored enhancement powder.

Don't let the little complexities involved in the nutrient control discourage you.

There was a time when foods could just be cooked up, canned or packaged and put on the store shelves with no indication of the contents or nutrients contained therein.

The Food and Drug Administration passed a law that every item packaged and sold has to have the contents listed in the "List of Ingredients" and that there has to be a "Nutrient facts" panel printed on the container.

The law has provided an exception for naturally occurring products, such as meats, vegetables and other foods that are not processed.

While the contents of the natural products are not required to have the same labeling rules as processed foods, the name and source of the natural products reflect the origins, such as meat labeling, that will have the "cut" identified. One example is the label for "Top Round Roast" verses "Bottom Round Roast", or "Shank".

The naming of different cuts of meat, for example, is designed to protect the consumer, but the bourdon of understanding of all of the terms is up to the consumer. There is no meat collage for this purpose. The naming requirements extend to all protein products.

At first, it took a lot of thought and a moderate amount of planning and discipline to check the "Nutrient Facts" panel on everything I buy, but now, I am finding that checking the

"Nutrient Facts" panel on everything I buy has become second nature to me. It just takes a bit of getting used to.

NO MORE MEAL LABELS

We are a product of our history. Phrases and ideas are carried forward through the decades even after they have lost their obvious value.

One such notion is the notion of "meal time". We eat because it is time to eat, not because we are hungry.

When it is not time to eat, we are taught to refrain from eating, such as the hours between dinner time and breakfast time.

The span of hours between the evening meal and the morning meal is very long. The body anticipates this fasting area in our day and causes you to want to fill the empty hours by snacking.

Abandon words like breakfast, lunch, dinner, supper, desert, snack, etc. These words define when it is time to eat and what types of foods are appropriate for the meal at this time of day. Your body could not care less what time it is.

I often eat what is considered to be a breakfast entree in the evening at a place that serves the "morning menu" all day long. It is high protein, low calorie and tends to fill you up, besides, (and this is the main reason) because it's allowed by my caloric intake plan and it just plain tastes good.

Eating what you want, when you want it, is one of the many benefits, while living on the quadrant plan. It really does not matter what you are eating, as long as the caloric content is in keeping with the program and the distribution of nutrients is correct.

If you eat a few more calories at one meal, you have to reduce the number of calories in the next meal to compensate.

Most of us, and I am no exception, break the rules and, midway between meals, will want to nibble on a few peanuts, popcorn or other snack food. Have the snack food on your list of favorite caloric items and remember to factor the calories in for these items.

When you have adjusted to the meals every 6 hours, you will find that 25 to 50 calories of snack food can take the edge off from your craving. Over time, your stomach naturally shrinks so that it only takes a tiny bit of munchies to stop your urge to snack.

In the event that you find yourself binge eating, when you are only trying to snack, then this is evidence of a possible food addiction and you should seek professional help from your Doctor, or a Nutritionist. If that is the case, this may not be the best plan for you if you are trying to reduce your body mass.

The number of total calories throughout the day must be limited to the allowance in the plan, or your weight loss goals will fail to materialize.

WEIGHT LOSS

Americans have recently become obsessed regarding the bodies proportions. Skinny runway models have destroyed the concept of healthy body proportions. Young girls are made to feel that they are fat, when they are normally proportioned.

If you want to lose weight, then decide how much you want to lose before you begin. Set a target weight. Be sensible about it. It's not healthy to conform to the standards imposed by Hollywood today.

I weighed in at 248 pounds and decided to reduce my weight to 185. That may seem to be a bit above the "recommended" weight, but I'm not going to be entering any beauty contest very soon.

If the weight is properly distributed, the body will appear pleasantly proportioned. The balance of fat to lean will be a better measure of my overall health than some blind number given on a chart.

Work out. Tone your muscles. Eat sensibly and monitor your weight. You will look and feel fine.

The BMI charts (Body Mass Index) are not the place to go for determining your ideal weight.

My ideal weight on the BMI chart is 150 pounds. I think that is too thin. Some reserve weight gives me a moderate level of comfort.

I want to be shapely without looking fat and at a weight that does not leave me looking lanky or skinny.

What is my beef with the traditional BMI charting system? Let me explain.

BMI, BODY MASS INDEX

There are metrics used in the health industry that are often not understood by the general public, such as BMI.

While some food choices may be beneficial to your general health and may help you to lose weight, some of the statistics around obesity have been falsely inflated to underscore the extent of the problem in America.

The BMI Chart is simple in its appearance and can raise the awareness of the problem in America to alarming statistical proportions. The fact is that the problem is not that severe.

The task of meeting the goal of a healthy body weight is not as difficult as it is portrayed to be.

It is easy to come to the conclusion that many health and nutrition experts are reaching far afield to convince the general public of the severity of the fitness problem in

America today. The general lack of overall fitness level with regard to Americans have been over exaggerated, to say the least.

The BMI Chart is a perfect example of this fact.

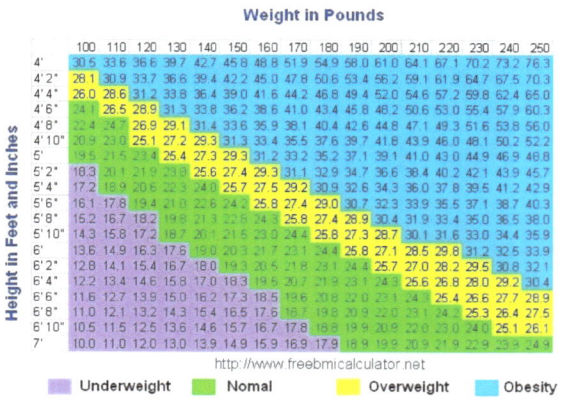

BMI is the height in inches plotted against the body weight of an individual without regard for the fat to lean content of the body mass.

A person can have a mere 10% body fat and be morbidly obese, according to the BMI index. Here are some examples:

1. Arnold Schwarzenegger, at the height of his bodybuilding career is rated as morbidly obese.

2. Body builders with their glistening skin and rippling muscular frames are rated as either obese, or morbidly obese.

3. Anyone with more than average muscular development may be rated as obese, because muscle tissue is far more dense and naturally weighs more than fat.

What percentage of Americans are truly obese? It isn't clear. There are fewer fat people in America than the statistic portrays because the statistic is flawed.

What can a little reserve do for you? Let me tell you a story about Lady and Girl.

I had two dogs. One was named Lady and the other was named Girl.

Lady was trim and well proportioned, while Girl was a bit chubby.

Both dogs contracted distemper and were under treatment by a Veterinarian. Both dogs were battling the disease and were losing weight at a steady pace.

My dog Lady, succumbed to the disease as she became so severely emaciated that she died. Meanwhile, Girl lost weight at about the same rate, but managed to recover. Although much thinner than her beginning weight, she was able to call upon her fat reserves to survive the ordeal during her recovery.

I'm not suggesting that you become, or remain fat. I am suggesting that you maintain a healthy, moderate reserve to call upon in the event of a life-threatening event.

WEIGHT MANAGEMENT

At first, weight management may seem to be a daunting task. That's only because the task is new and it takes a bit of getting used to. You notice that we don't talk about "diet" in the context of unpleasant eating restrictions.

A diet, in the most recognizable form, is a desperate, but temporary resolution to an alarming problem. You may think that if you only could lose the weight, it would fix everything.

Remember the complex distribution of nutrients discussed in the chapter, "Nutrient Distribution"?

Do not attempt to solve the problem of balancing your diet during the early phases of your weight loss.

Nutrient distribution is a problem that you can resolve later on. For now, take it easy and take it slow.

Plot a steady course by focusing on caloric intake and when you are happy with your appearance, refocus on improving your choice of foods so that you can fine-tune your nutrient needs.

The sad fact remains that the weight is not the problem. The weight is merely an outward symptom that manifests itself. The problem is your caloric intake, not your body mass.

The outward manifestation of body mass causes us, and others, to see what is believed to be the entire dilemma, and therefore, the cause. The real solution is masked by our horror regarding what we see. So we diet.

The solution is to change our attitude regarding our goal.

The solution is clear. We stop "Dieting" in the classic sense. We simply regulate our food intake. Regulating our food intake results in the body naturally assuming the pleasing proportions that nature intended.

You are not "on a diet". You are modifying you're eating habits and an adjustment in body mass naturally follows. Focus on eating well, with sensible portions, not on losing weight.

Once your body naturally achieves its goal weight, weigh often, perhaps weekly, at the same time of the day and weight gain will never sneak up on you again. You need not be obsessed regarding your weight. You need only be aware of it.

I vividly remember the mornings when I had to suck in my stomach in order to button my pants. The problem was obviously caused by using hot water to launder my pants. They were shrinking in the wash, or maybe in the dryer. Who knew which?

Then one day the realization struck me, that the pants just never seemed to stop shrinking and I had to but new pants.

Isn't it odd though? I never seemed to notice that my belt was shrinking too. I was blind to the problem until it was completely out of control.

If you adjust your daily caloric intake to bring your weight under control when a problem is first detected. You will find weight management to be easier than discovering, to your surprise, that your pants do not button easily any more.

BALANCE AND MODERATION

I am not a Mormon, but the Mormons have what they refer to as "the word of wisdom". The word of wisdom is "moderation in all things". Contrary to popular belief, it does not come from the "Bible" or "The Book of Mormon" neither does it come from their book, "The Pearl of Great Prize". While there may be several quotes regarding "temperance", the word of wisdom, while good advice, was created in its verbatim form, by the Mormons. I digress.

The word of wisdom is a guide to living that makes good sense, especially in terms of diet. You can eat anything you want, any time you want, in moderation. Your total end of the day calories, protein, fat and other nutrient count is what matters.

If you have 100 calories more than you should in the morning, then you have to reduce the caloric intake by the end of the day by 100 to account for it, which would require a decrease from 500 calories to only 400, for example.

If you have no protein in the midday meal, then the protein count for the other 3 meals have to increase to make up for it.

In this way, you can enjoy a snack or a treat with friends once in a while. Special events, such as birthdays, Christmas or Thanksgiving celebrations need not be a problem. Just do not start believing that a party once in a while won't matter. It may not, but it will be the beginning of your ride down that slippery slope, where you wonder why your pants do not fit any more. Your clothes are not shrinking in the wash.

The best way to ensure balance and moderation is to buy and consume fresh foods in far greater proportions than canned goods.

Try not to open more than two or three cans a week and make sure that they are not heavy laden with fat and calories.

On the subject of retaining a balancing of all the nutrients, such as fat, protein and carbohydrates, the best you can do is count calories and eat fresh, natural foods.

You should always have a protein and a carbohydrate. Fats are needed to some degree, but getting 25 to 30 percent fat is less important than the other nutrients. As long as you get fats and they are less than 30% of the calories in your meal you are doing fine.

FULLER, MORE JOYFUL LIVING

Just to recap, when you eat right, you have more energy, become sick less often and feel great.

When you change your diet by dividing your day into quadrants, you never get too hungry before it's meal time again.

This is a lifestyle change. Not a weight loss diet. You can lose weight far more easily using this method and ease into painless weight management mode when your target weight is achieved.

This allows you to have four good meals a day and distribute the calories, carbs, protein and fats across more meals for a fuller, more satisfying meal opportunity.

This removes meal labels and gives you total flexibility with regard to meal content.

Take charge of your diet. Create weight loss and maintain normal weight more effectively while eating more of the foods you enjoy most.

While you are losing that weight, if weight was a problem, do not sit on the couch. You can naturally watch the TV shows that you love, but make sure you venture outside every day. Go somewhere. Do something, anything to get out of the house and breathe fresh air.

Getting outside will help you to reduce your desire to snack, because you will not be near snack foods.

The change of scenery will help you to put your mind elsewhere. Social interaction will enable you to get outside of yourself psychologically.

Take up a hobby, join a club. Keep moving to keep your mind occupied. Over time you will become accustomed to being on the move. Being outside on a daily basis will make you restless when you have to stay inside. Life will become richer for the experience.

My experience is that while I like to get out and keep moving, it is not a good idea to eat out. Restaurant foods contain unknown ingredients and may contain quantities of additives and preservatives due to the lack of fresh ingredients.

Restaurants do not care about nutrition. They are in the business of selling food to as many people each day as possible.

They make the food taste good, no matter what ingredients and no matter in what proportions, in order to bring people back.

HOW DOES THIS AFFECT DIABETICS?

If you heeded the advice in the chapter, "Introduction" and again, in the chapter, "The Quadrant Method" good for you. Now, if you are diabetic, I recommend that you seek the advice of your Doctor of Pharmacy and/or your Endocrinologist.

I remind you again, that I am not a Physician and the content of this book, and especially this chapter, is a calorie control method that has worked for me, with some additional considerations.

This book applies to you, but, as with me, there is more to know if you happen to be diabetic.

The life of the diabetic is complicated, because you have to supplement the control of calories with the simultaneous control of your blood sugar.

There are two types of diabetes;

There is type 1, for those who are born with the inability to manufacture insulin.

There is type 2, or "Adult onset diabetes, for those who acquire a resistance to insulin. They are very different.

These differences between types of diabetes are the reason that it is imperative that you consult a medical professional that is qualified to respond to any questions regarding this book.

I say this, not out of any "cover your butt" motive. I truly warn you, when it comes to the methods and experience in this book, check it out. Especially the experiences and information shared in this chapter.

NOW, ON WITH THE INFORMATION

Whether you are using pills to regulate your blood sugar, or insulin, always check your blood sugar.

I have a glucometer and test strips and check my blood sugar four times a day. I test it each quadrant just before eating the quadrant meal.

As you reduce, or regulate your caloric intake, you may notice that there is a tendency to "crash".

When you crash, your blood sugar levels will fall until you become weak, dizzy, sweaty, and shaky. If untreated, you will eventually lose consciousness. Unless you take something in order to raise your blood sugar to normal, you could die.

Normal blood sugar level is ideally 100 milligrams per deciliter.

In addition to counting calories, I strongly recommend that you also count carbohydrates.

All carbohydrates contain calories, but not all calories contain carbohydrates.

The important task is to ad those calories in the carbohydrates to the calories that do not have carbohydrates.

If your goal is 350 calories. You may have Scali bread at 100 calories and 24 grams, along with sardines at 200 calories and 0 grams of carbohydrates, followed by a tangerine at 47 calories and 12 grams of carbohydrates.

If we break it down;

Food Item	calories	carbs
Scali bread	100	24
Sardines	200	0
Tangerine	47	12
TOTALS	347	36

The 350 calorie requirement is met with 347 calories. This meal is short by three calories, but will be close enough to our goal.

The 36 carbohydrate total will dictate how many units of fast acting insulin, possibly Humalog, that we need to inject.

If your doctor told you to take 1 unit of insulin for every 12 carbohydrates, then your shot dosage would be 3 units.

Body chemistry is a complex thing, but the difference between (carbohydrates), carbs and calories is simple.

Insulin will lower your blood sugar.

Carbs will raise your blood sugar.

Calories will increase your weight.

Any blood sugar that is not burned, when combined with insulin, is stored as fat. The calorie is a unit measure of energy.

The calorie is defined as the energy needed to increase the temperature of 1 gram of water by 1 degree centigrade.

So, you see, a calorie is not a thing. It's a unit of heat energy. The heat energy is derived from carbohydrates that raise the level of glucose (blood sugar).

Carbohydrates are any of a large group of organic compounds occurring in foods and living tissues and including sugars, starch, and cellulose. They contain hydrogen and oxygen in the same ratio as water (2:1) and typically can be broken down to release energy (calories) in the human body.

Are you confused yet? Not to worry, it is only given here as nice to know information. It is not important to know this, just be aware of your calorie, carb, and insulin requirements.

With regard to jogging or working out, be very careful when on a reduced calorie intake regimen. You blood sugar is more likely to dip below normal and you could crash.

Make sure to keep some form of candy close at hand in case your blood sugar unexpectedly drops too low.

When you start to decrease your caloric intake, at first, enter into your exercise routine gradually, until you get a feel for how your body is going to react.

When I started out on my exercise routines, I took care to ensure that my workout time was the same each day.

I also took care to ensure that my meal preceding the workout was as close to the same every time.

Also, make sure your blood sugar levels are the same and that your medication does not vary, but always conforms to your Doctors instructions.

~~~ THE END ~~~

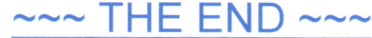

www.ingramcontent.com/pod-product-compliance
Lightning Source LLC
Chambersburg PA
CBHW050845290526
45792CB00002B/522